The Textbook of The Non-Medical Prescribing Journey is a true representation of a nurses' journey through university on the Non-Medical Prescribing course.

It is easy-to-read, and delivers key points to help comprehend all the essential knowledge required to succeed on the course.

It discusses key issues and skills relevant to non-medical prescribing. Now fully updated and linked to the National Prescribing Centre Single Competency Framework for non-medical prescribers.

It shows activities to help you link your continuing professional development within the competences required as a prescriber and revalidation.

This practical title remains an ideal resource for all qualified health professionals to practice safe and effective non-medical prescribing.

The core themes are pharmacodynamics, pharmacokinetics, prescribing principles, and continuing professional development. It sets out 2 university assignments which passed and can be used as guidance for course work. It focuses on contraception and diabetes.

Key Features:

- Accessible and study-friendly

  Written by a Community Specialist Practitioner, RGN, Practice Nurse

- The story of a true journey on the Non-Medical Prescribing course

- learning objectives and activities to support a deeper understanding of the theoretical knowledge base and its application to practice

- Case studies linking the topics to real-life scenarios

  The Textbook of Non-Medical Prescribing provides support to anyone studying for a prescribing qualification or looking for a refresher on the subject.

Drug Metabolism

Lipid soluble agents are metabolized to water soluble compounds. This aids excretion by the kidney. Some drugs can induce the drug metabolizing enzyme. Some drugs need to be metabolized before they can be pharmacologically active. Some "active drugs also have active metabolites. Some drugs have metabolites which are toxic.

First Pass Metabolism

Can be explained as the first time the drug reaches the liver following oral absorption. The drug is absorbed and reaches the liver via the hepatic portal system.

Some drugs undergo extensive 1st pass metabolism when they reach the liver. Hence the reason we do not give some drugs orally. Examples of these drugs would be imipramine, morphine, propranolol, buprenorphine, diazepam, midazolam, demerol, cimetidine, and lidocaine.

When the drug reaches the liver the concentration of a drug is greatly reduced before it reaches circulation. During first pass metabolism, the following will occur oxidation, reduction and hydrolysis of the drug.

So, first pass metabolism is transformation of a drug into a more polar metabolite. A process whereby the concentration of a drug is greatly reduced before it reaches the systemic circulation. It is the fraction of drug lost during the process of absorption. First pass metabolism reduces the bioavailability of a drug.

Second Pass Metabolism

During second pass metabolism, the drug undergoes conjugation. This is the second time the drug passes through the liver. Conjugation occurs entirely in the liver. The process involves a combination of a glucuronic, sulphuric, acetic, amino acid with a functioning group to form polar conjugate.

Bioavailability

Can be explained as the proportion of the administered dose which reaches circulation unchanged. It is the percentage or fraction of the drug which is available in the circulatory system. Or can be explained as the proportion of the drug that reaches systemic circulation unaltered. As previously discussed first pass metabolism greatly reduces bioavailability.

This means the oral dose is taken and then some is destroyed in the gut, and not absorbed. Some is destroyed by gut wall. Some is destroyed by the liver. The remaining dose gets to systemic circulation.

Bioequivalent

Can means that 2 drug products have the same percentage of active ingredient. It therefore has the same rate and extent of absorption. Bioequivalence is a term in pharmacokinetics used to assess the expected in vivo BIOLOGICAL EQUIVALENCE of two proprietary preparations of a drug. If two products are said to be BIOEQUIVALENT it MEANS that they would be expected to be, for all intents and purposes, the same.

Note – The significance is that we would never prescribe generically when we need a drug to be bioequivalent. Some drugs must be bioequivalent. Meaning we must never prescribe them generically.

For example, epileptic drugs. The proportion of the drug differs with generic prescribing. Therefore, the drug would not have the same effect under generic prescribing.

The Phases of licensing a medicine

1. The use of small scale volunteers.

2. The dose must be established

3. Large Scale Clinical Trials are conducted

4. Pharmacovigilance.

   Volunteers will agree to participate in the small-scale trials. The trials are usually males as obviously, they have no risk of pregnancy. Once the dosage has been established to trial, then large clinical scale trials are planned and conducted.

   These trials are double blinded trials, meaning neither the nurse or health practitioner conducting the trial or the volunteer knows whether they have received the drug or a placebo. Pharmacovigilance then needs to be applied. This means that we must be vigilant and report any adverse effects or side effects on the yellow card system either by the cards in the BNF or online.

   Black triangle warning must be applied, where we inform of anything and we send any information to MHRA to identify and problems or safety issues.

An Unlicensed Medication

Can be explained as a drug which does not hold a marketing authorization in this country. Note – Mixing of drugs makes them unlicensed. When a drug is put in a syringe driver for example and mixed with another substance or drug it is then unlicensed use simply because it has now been mixed.

Unlicensed Use

Is when the drug holds a marketing authorization, but you use the drug outside this authorization.

NOTE – examples would be Levonelle used up to 5 days' post pregnancy risk, but its marketing authorization is 72 hours' post pregnancy risk.

Another example would be Metformin tablets used in polycystic ovary, because although Metformin is used for polycystic ovary treatment its marketing authorization if for use with Diabetes.

Adverse Drug Reaction

Any drug can produce unwanted or unexpected adverse reactions. Rapid detection and recording of adverse drug reaction is of vital importance so that unrecognized hazards are identified promptly. Then appropriate steps can be taken to ensure the safety of this drug.

Can be described as an unwanted, harmful reaction in man with a normal dose. There are 2 types of drug reaction type A and B.

Type A = predictable, generally don't cause harm.

Type B = Rare, with a high mortality rate, can be fatal.

Note – The reason why newly licensed drugs are intentionally monitored. Newly licensed drugs all have a black triangle warning. This means we want more information about these drugs and the black triangle can be seen as a warning sign to report any incidents of side effects etc.

Agonist and antagonists

Any drug, chemical or ligand which can interact with a receptor can cause or inhibit a biological response in the body. These can be split into 2 groups agonist and antagonist.

AGONIST

Is a chemical, drug or ligand that binds to a receptor and activates the receptor to produce a biological response. An example would be Morphine

ANTAGONIST

Is a chemical, drug, or ligand that binds to a receptor and blocks a response. An example would be Naloxone.

There are other examples and it is important you learn more about these other examples. Smoking and smoking cessation drugs are another example.

Pro-Drugs

Can be explained as a compound that is itself biologically inactive. To become active, it needs to undergo metabolism in the liver. Lipid lowering statins are one example of a pro-drug. Another example is prednisolone.

Narrow Therapeutic Window Drugs

These drugs have a narrow window between been therapeutic and toxic.

Examples of these drugs are digoxin and lithium, theophylline. The use of these drugs requires monitoring of bloods at regular intervals to ensure the safety of the user.

Advisory Drug Labels

All drugs have certain advisory labels relevant to their use and administration.

POM = Prescription Only Medicines

P= Pharmacy Medicines

GSL = General Sales List

P medicines have a different license than a POM i.e. Levonelle sold over the counter.

SLS = selected list scheme (means this can be given on the NHS)

The structure of the cell

The cell structure is made of phosphor lipid. Fat soluble material, pass through cell membrane easily. Hence most drugs are lipid soluble. Sodium flows out the cell and potassium flows in. Cells have a membrane a nucleus and cytoplasm. Receptors will sit on the membrane of the cell. When cells are lipid soluble they glide across the membrane easily. When cells are water soluble they require a secondary messenger to assist in the process.

Secondary Messenger Mechanism

Secondary Cell messengers provide a way of relaying a message from outside the cell inside the cell, when the cell is water soluble. This is a complex process to understand and hopefully can be easily understood when explained as follows: -

1. A hormone locks onto the receptor.

2. This then activates the G protein.

3. The G Protein then shifts across

4. This activates Adenosynetryphosphate (ALP) which is already in the cell.

5. When (ALP) is activated it converts to Cyclic Adenosine monophosphate (CAMP).

6. (CAMP) is the secondary messenger and turn things on and off.

7. Whilst this is happening Calcium comes rushing in through the channel and switches on the Enzyme called Phosphodiesterase.

8. (CAMP) is broken down by this.

9. So, the mechanism is making (CAMP) and breaking it down.

10. This process STOPS only when the hormone wither detaches or goes deep into the cell and lays dormant.

An example of this process is glucose and insulin.

For a secondary messenger to work effectively it must have amplification and control specificity. Note Caffeine inhibits the breakdown of CAMP.

Functions of Membranes

Membranes have many functions. They protect the cell. They guard incoming and outgoing substances. They maintain Ion concentration. They regulate by being permeable keeping some cells in and letting others out. For example, potassium and sodium, of in the kidney large molecules are kept in and small ones out.

Blood brain barrier

The blood brain barrier allows some substances into the brain but screens out toxins and bacteria. Some substances that are allowed to cross are waters, co2, o2, amino acids, alcohol and antihistamine. Some infections that are allowed to cross the blood brain barrier are HIV and bacterial meningitis.

Methods of transfusion across membranes

1. Diffusion – the substance passes from a level of high concentration to low concentration.

2. Osmosis – the movement of water requires a cell membrane.

3. Facilitated Diffusion

4. Active Transport

Hypertonic solution - one solution has higher concentration than the other.

Isotonic - both solutions have same concentration.

The Inflammatory Response

The inflammatory response is a healing mechanism. It is the body's response to damage. Damage will occur due to infection or heat or trauma. During the inflammatory response key things are happening in the immune system such as changes in the cell, vasodilation and diapedesis.

There are mechanisms around the capillaries to stop it happening. The capillaries are made of endothelial cells. The blood vessels are lined with these. The Endothelial cells are the only surface that blood comes into contact with and remain fluid. Endothelial cells can also tell the body that there is a virus.

Histamine receptors sit on endothelial cell walls. When the cells become damaged histamine is released from the mast cells. When the histamine is released from the mast cells, the histamine causes the smooth muscle to relax.

Neutrophils then move by a process of margination and they stick to the cell wall. Neutrophils then look for holes to get through and when they find one they get through. This process is called diapedesis. When the neutrophils leave the cell water and electrolytes also leave. During diapedesis antibiotics and clotting proteins can leave also. Red blood cells do not leave the cells.

The leaving of neutrophils, water, electrolytes, clotting proteins and antibiotics etc. creates a fibrin mesh,

The fibrin mesh traps debris and infection.

Mediators in the inflammatory response

Histamine – is released from the mast cells
Leukotrienes and prostaglandins come along and produce a response.

Leukotrienes and prostaglandins can be manufactured in stressed cells.

Prescribing in Pregnancy

Drugs can harm the fetus **at any time** during pregnancy. It is important to understand the effects drugs may cause at each trimester.

1st trimester – drugs may cause congenital malformations **during weeks 3-11 of 40.**

2nd and 3rd trimester – Drugs may affect the growth and functional development.

Most important to remember If you don't need it don't give it!!

Always refer to the British National Formulary (BNF) latest edition as this will show you the drugs that are deemed harmful in pregnancy and the drugs that are not harmful in pregnancy. If in doubt do not prescribe and seek specialist advice from General Practitioner or consultant.

Consider the following: -

1. Teratogenesis effect is the toxic effect of the drug.

2. Will it cross the barrier i.e. placenta or milk?

3. Which trimester are they in?

4. Metabolism of both mother & fetus.

5. Will the drug create a metallic taste in the milk?

6. The molecular size and weight will play a part in whether it crosses the placenta.

7. Exposure, duration, dose, route, iv or oral, fetal metabolism, maternal illness.

Tetrogenic

Tetrogenic means a drug or substance which causes fetal malformations, abnormalities in physiological or mental development or impairment of growth and development. Remember drugs in the environment such as tobacco, carbon monoxide are environmental risks.

Prescribing in Breast feeding

When prescribing in breast feeding consider the following:

1. The therapeutic effect in mother and the unwanted effect in child.

2. The extent of transfer of drug into milk – usually only 1-2% of total maternal dose is transferred to the infant.

3. Most drugs cause no effect to breast fed baby or infant.

4. Chemotherapy, high dose estrogens, high dose vitamin D, lithium.

5. Is the drug necessary?

6. Is it safe?

7. Could a sustained release/slow acting drug be used?

8. If there is a high risk should you measure serum levels in the infant?

9. What are the side effects for both mum and infant?

Prescribing in Children

Firstly, remember all medication for children is listed in the British National Formulary (BNF) for children.

When prescribing for children always refer to the children's (BNF) latest edition,

A child is aged between 1 – 12.

An adolescent is 12+ years.

Always consider the adverse drug reactions in children.

Take care in writing the prescription and note the child's age also.

Be vigilant to consider all aspects such as rare pediatric conditions, dosage in children, dose calculation, dose frequency.

Take care to ensure there is no hepatic or renal impairment in the child.

Absorption, metabolism and distribution altered in children this is decreased. This is due to immaturity of gut, liver and kidneys.

Drugs are prescribed based on weight and up to date weights must be obtained at each visit or prescribing assessment.

Cytochrome P450 Enzyme System

The cytochrome P450 enzymes (CYP), are a family of enzymes which live primarily in the liver and small intestine. The cytochrome P450 (CYP) mixed function monooxygenases, are located on the smooth endoplasmic reticulum of cells throughout the body.

They will either inhibit or enhance the effect of a drug. They also function to metabolize toxic compounds. Cytochrome P450 enzymes will either act as **Inhibitors** when they will make drugs work slower and for longer. Fluoxetine is an inhibitor. Inhibitors increase the effects on the body of drugs.

The cytochrome P450 enzymes also work as Inducers when they will make drugs work faster and for a shorter time. Examples of substances that works as inhibitors on the body are smoking and grapefruit juice.

These enzymes are responsible for the oxidative (Phase 1) metabolism of a wide number of compounds, including many medications. The play a role in in drug interactions, drug toxicity, and the creation of carcinogenic by products.

There are many types of (CYP) within the family but CYP 3A4 AND CYP 2D6 are the 2 enzymes associated with drug interactions and side effects.

Xenobiotics

Some xenobiotics cause toxicity by disrupting normal cell function. They bind and damage proteins, DNA and Lipids. They react in the cell with oxygen to form free radicals, which damage lipid, protein and DNA. We are exposed to a great number of xenobiotics during our lifetime. Xenobiotics – can be pharmaceuticals and food components. A xenobiotic is a foreign chemical substance, not normally found and our body detoxifies them.

The body detoxifies them as we have evolved complex systems of detoxification enzymes. These enzymes function adequately to minimize the potential of damage from xenobiotics. Parkinson's disease and chronic fatigue/immune dysfunction syndrome are associated with impaired detoxification. Mutations in P450 cytochrome enzymes are responsible for several human diseases. They can convert pro-carcinogens to carcinogens

Enzymes

Enzymes are catalytic proteins.
Enzymes increase reaction from thousands to millions of time faster from the uncatalyzed state. Enzymes allow metabolism to occur.

Mechanisms that promote drug clearance by the kidney

The kidneys are responsible primarily for the control of blood pressure, filtration, secretion and re-absorption. Filtration occurs within the glomerulus. Secretion occurs as the kidney secrete drugs bound to protein and excrete them. Re-absorption, happens in the distal portion of the nephron. OCTS and OATS – are attaching to give a negative or positive charge. Many arterials feed into the glomerulus, with an in and out gate, causing filtration. The large molecules such as blood proteins are kept inside the kidney and the small molecules such as electrolytes are excreted.

The GUT

The structures of the gut are firstly a high surface area. The gut has a rich blood supply. Within the gut are many plica, 600 folds and pockets, along with villi and micro villi. The function of the gut is to mix things up, by churning them and adding enzymes to the contents to break it down. The mixing of the contents enhances absorption, allowing the food to trickle through the small intestine.

Neurotransmission

Neurotransmitters are the brain chemicals that communicate information throughout our brain and body. They relay signals between nerve cells, called "neurons."

The brain uses neurotransmitters to tell your heart to beat, your lungs to breathe, and your stomach to digest. They can also affect mood, sleep, concentration, weight, and can cause adverse symptoms when they are out of balance.
Neurotransmitter levels can be depleted many ways.

There are two kinds of neurotransmitters 1. Inhibitory and 2. excitatory. Excitatory neurotransmitters stimulate the brain. Inhibitory neurotransmitters calm the brain and help create balance. Examples of neurotransmitters are Adrenaline and Serotonin. Serotonin is an inhibitory neurotransmitter which means that it does not stimulate the brain. Adequate amounts of serotonin are necessary for a stable mood and to balance any excessive excitatory (stimulating) neurotransmitter firing in the brain.

If you use stimulant medications or caffeine in your daily regimen, it can cause a depletion of serotonin over time. Serotonin also regulates many other processes such as carbohydrate cravings, sleep cycle, pain control and appropriate digestion.

Adrenalin on the other hand is an excitatory neurotransmitter that is reflective of stress. This neurotransmitter will often be elevated when ADHD like symptoms are present. Long term stress or insomnia can cause epinephrine levels to be depleted low. Adrenaline also regulates our heart rate and blood pressure.

Surface Cell Receptors

Cell surface receptors are **receptors** at the surface of a **cell** (built into its **cell membrane**) that act in a **cell signaling** by receiving (binding to) extracellular **molecules**. They are specialized **integral membrane proteins** that allow communication between the cell and the outside world.

The extracellular molecules may be **hormones, neurotransmitters, cytokines, growth factors, cell adhesion molecules**, or nutrients. They react with the receptor to induce changes in the **metabolism** and activity of a cell. In the process of **signal transduction**, **ligand** binding affects a cascading chemical change through the cell membrane.

Hormones and Receptors

Hormones are chemical messengers. They are either water of fat soluble. Hormones interact with receptor molecules and switch mechanisms on or off. In order that a chemical qualify as a hormone it must fulfil the 3 points: -

1. It must be released in its active form.

2. It must be delivered to its target cells by the blood.

3. When it reaches, its target cell the chemical must interact with a receptor on or within the target cell.

If a chemical fails on one of these criteria it does not qualify as a hormone. A hormone can also be referred to as the first messenger. The level of activity of a hormone at the target cell is determined by the follow: -

1. The concentrate of the hormone in the blood.

2. The receptor binding affinity of the hormone.

3. The number of receptor sites occupied.

4. The duration of the binding, and the receptor population number on, or in, the target cell.

Examples of hormones are testosterone, estrogen, follicle stimulating hormone (FSH) and Luteinizing hormone (LH).

If hormones are fat soluble they glide through the cell. If hormones are water soluble they need a secondary messenger mechanism. Water soluble hormones interact with cell surface receptors.

What is a receptor

A protein which binds a first messenger and is involved in mediating its biological effects is known as a receptor. Most receptors it seems are located on the outside of the cell, and thus signal transduction occurs through the membrane. Receptor numbers can go up or down. Cells can gain or lose receptors. Thus, they can be more or less responsive.

All cells must engage in some form of communication which permits the cells to interact with the environment within the body. Isolated cells die. Intercellular communication must be maintained in order to prevent cells undergoing apoptosis.

Nervous system

At the synapse the presynaptic terminal secretes neurotransmitter chemicals such as acetylcholine and serotonin. In addition, several neuromodulators can be released by this terminal to influence the postsynaptic dendrite.

Endocrine system

A number of well defined, glandular structures produce and secrete chemical messengers called hormones. Each hormone has its own specificity and therefore has an inductive effect a predetermined range of target cells.

Immune System

Cells of the immune system produce a coordinated attack on non-self-antigens. These cells communicate using a variety of chemical messengers such as leukotrienes and interleukins.

Half Life - Can be described as the time taken for plasma concentration to half.

Plasma protein and drugs

A drug when bound to plasma protein is inactive. Only free drug is biologically active.

Drug metabolism and its stages in the body

1. Absorption

2. Metabolism

3. Distribution

4. Elimination

   Absorption is concerned with what happens to the drug once it is taken orally and how it is absorbed in the gut. Metabolism occurs within the liver. There are 2 stages first pass and second pass. Distribution is how the drug travels around the body in the blood stream.
   Elimination is how the body excretes the drug i.e. in the urine, faeces or breast milk etc.

   ## Generic Prescribing

   Is the recommended best practice when prescribing a drug? However, some drugs must be bioequivalent and we must pay attention to this for example epileptic drugs.

   The reason we prescribe generically is predominantly due to cost. Generic drugs are cheaper than the brand. To understand this thing of Heinz beans as the brand and Asda's beans as the generic. A list of reason we prescribe generically: -

1. It saves time.
2. There is a good supply of generic medication available.
3. The BNF has a section on generic prescribing.
4. It is good practice.
5. It is cost effective.
6. It is policy.
7. It will reduce prescribing costs on the budget.

Examples of generic prescribing are: -

Prescribe Desogestrel (generic) instead of Cerazette (brand).

Prescribe Rigevidon (generic) instead of Microgynon (brand)

The biggest barrier to generic prescribing is often the patient as they are often saying well that is not as good as Cerazette or Microgynon. In these instances, we must justify our practice to satisfy our clients.

Supplementary Prescribing

In the application of supplementary prescribing it is the Doctor or Dentist who has full responsibility for the drugs being prescribed. It involves an agreed plan of care by several practitioners and of course the patient themselves.

It requires specific agreement. The patient is involved in the decisions and the agreement. There will be a written agreed documented care plan and clinical management plan. A template is useful to fulfil the criteria.

There must be structure with clear directions. This will be structured to make it patient specific. Guidelines and protocols must be considered and followed.

The Liver

As we already know the liver is responsible for metabolisation of drugs.

Phase 1 – Oxygen added this acts as a hook.
Phase 2 – Oxygen that hooks a conjugate.

These two phases – convert a fat-soluble drug to a lipid soluble compound to a water-soluble compound.

Phase 2 metabolism involves CONJUGATION - that is, the attachment of an ionized ... forming a range of ionized metabolites that CAN then be excreted in the urine.

Water soluble compounds are excreted through the kidneys.

Controlled Drugs

The Misuse of Drugs ACT (1971) prohibits certain activities in relation to 'controlled drugs'. It is illegal to manufacture, supply or possess these drugs. The offences applicable are graded according to the class of the drug. Prescriptions for these drugs have legal requirements as stated below.

If you intend to prescribe these when qualified as a Non-Medical Prescriber, be vigilant in the prescription requirements, instalments and repeats, private prescriptions, Department of Health Guidance (DOH), dependence and misuse, supervised consumption, prescribing drugs likely to cause dependence or misuse and travelling abroad.

In England doctors, should report when they are providing structured treatment for substance dependence to their local National Drug Treatment Monitoring System (NDTMS) Team. Note the most serious drugs of addiction are cocaine, diamorphine hydrochloride (heroin) and synthetic opioids.

Legal requirements for controlled drugs

A prescription for a controlled drug must state the following: -

1. Drug

2. Strength

3. 3. Directions for use

4. Quantity in word and figures.

NMP LEGISLATION AND THE IMPACT ON YOU

Medicines Act (1968)

Misuse of Drug Act (1971)

Misuse of Drugs Amendment in (2006) meant all nurses able to prescribe wider

Prescriptions by Nurses (1992)

Health & Social Care Act (2001)

Health Act (2003)

Medicines Act (1968) was replaced by Human

Medicines Regulations (2012)
The impact of this on the practitioner is <u>that</u> you need to demonstrate what has enabled you to prescribe. How can you prove your competence within any area?

Misuse of Drugs Act (2001)

Schedule 2

Covers drugs such as (Opiates such as Pethidine Diamorphine and Methadone)

Schedule 3

Covers drugs such as (Barbiturates, Tramadol, Temgesic and Temazepam)

Schedule 4 part 1

Covers drugs such as (Benzodiazepines, Tranquilizers, Nitrazepam, Diazepam and Lorazepam)

Schedule 4 part 2

Covers drugs such as (Anabolic and Androgenic steroids)

Schedule 5

Covers drugs such as (Codeine, Oramorph, Folcadene cough mixture and Dihydrocoedine)

SYMBOLS IN THE BNF AND WHAT DO THEY MEAN

At the side of each drugs there are symbols such as a round black circle this refers to the side effects of the drug. There may be a black triangle see chemotherapy drugs for this is common there.

Black triangle is a warning that if side effects occur these must be reported to the Medicines healthcare and Regulatory Products Agency (MHRA). This information is stored and if repeat side effects or ill consequences arising then the (MHRA) can see this is a problem and a risk to the public. This should stop tragedies such as the Thalidomide disaster, when side effects of a drug caused deformed limbs and this went unnoticed for a long time.

PACT DATA

This is a term you will hear a lot. It stands for Prescribing Analyst and Audit Information. In simple terms, it means you are being monitored with all your prescribing electronically.

When a prescription is produced by either a General Practitioner or any other prescriber, the contents of the same is recorded. Then audit is carried out to establish things such as the frequency of all drugs been prescribed. The cost of that individual prescriber's prescriptions is recorded. This is all available and stored for future reference. This data would hopefully identify an untoward prescribe practices and again it ensures safety and good practice with prescribing. Thing of this when you prescribe we are all accountable for everything we prescribe and the cost and generic prescribing are our priority as practitioners.

Pharmacokinetics

Pharmacokinetics is simply concerned with how the drug moves through the body and what the body does to the drug. So, from swallowing the drug orally what then does the body do with the same. Consider it as the movement of the drug from going in to leaving the body. The body absorbs the drug, metabolizes the drug, distributes it and finally excretes the same.

Absorption

Metabolism

Distribution

Excretion

Absorption occurs in the gut and metabolism in the liver. Plasma protein plays a role in distribution of the drug. For distribution drugs have to bind to plasma protein. So, if the person has less plasma protein for example then the distribution will be affected. It makes sense then if the person has more plasma protein then the drug will be distributed more rapidly.

When thinking about pharmacokinetics, we must consider: -

1. What happens to this patient?

2. What will happen to the serum and plasma?

3. What will happen to the kidneys?

4. What will happen to the liver?

Pharmacodynamics

Pharmacodynamics on the other hand is simply about the biochemical and physiological effects of drugs on the body. So, what the drug does to the body. It is about the dynamics of the drug. This involves receptor binding. It involves chemical reactions. Thing of pharmacodynamics as the relationship between the dose and response, i.e., the drug's effects. The pharmacologic response depends on the drug binding to its target.

The Cell

Human body made us of 3 components

1. Cells

2. Fibres

3. Matrix

   Cells determine our structure. They rule our biochemistry and our metabolism. Cells have a nucleus and a cytoplasm. Any material found outside the nucleus is termed the cytoplasm. The functions of the cell are synthesized by materials called enzymes. Enzymes help to regulate energy production, synthesis and breakdown within the cell. There are 46 chromosomes. These are 2 sets of 23. These cells in a human are made up 23 from paternal (father) and 23 from maternal (mother). Each chromosome is made up of a mix of DNA and RNA and proteins.

Prescriptions

All prescriptions are valid for 6 months from the date of issue unless they are a controlled drug or substance.

A prescription for a controlled drug is valid for 28 days from the date of issue.

If the CD requires dispensing in instalments the first dose must be prescribed within 28 days of the issue date otherwise it is no longer valid.

Black triangle drugs

These are generally drugs that are new on the market. They have a marketing authorization, but the (MHRA) need more information. Think newly licensed, new risks, and report anything the patient advises you or you notice as been a side effect, ill effect or significantly unusual.

You can report to the MHRA directly on line at **www.MHRA.co.uk** or you can report using the yellow cards in the back of the BNF.

Remember if in doubt report and that it is best to report than not report. Report anything.

Double blinded placebo multi-site randomized trial

These are the large clinical trials that are play a role in the licensing process of any drug. Remember the practitioner giving the drugs and the volunteer remain unaware if they have had the drug or the placebo. They can then be deemed randomized, double blinded and have rigor as evidence and research. We can be confident in the findings using this process. They are completed on multi-sites by multiple practitioners and volunteers. The placebo affect remains unknown and is vital in these trials.

Types of muscle in the body

There are 3 types of muscle in the body which are cardiac, skeletal and smooth. If we mess around and interfere with the calcium (Ca+) level, you will affect the smooth muscle found in the gut.

Enzymes

Enzymes play many roles they can: -

    a) break something down
b) make something bigger & better
c) they can change something

Remember, enzymes do not break drugs now and you should never suggest they do. There are over 30 enzymes in the P450 system.

However, two of these are the most important CYP 3A4 AND CYP 2D6. These 2 have been identified over recent years as the two that cause many of the side effects and interactions we see from medication.

Much has still to be learnt about why, never the less it is fact these are the CYP enzymes which do cause the majority of the problems.

Examples of Prescribing Logs

We have talked a lot about what we must consider when we are going to issue a prescription. Now let us look at some template examples of prescribing in practice and how this was considered and assessed and what the outcome was. Remember this is an in-depth process where many factors are considered, the client or patient is involved in the process. Once a prescription is issued it is noted that a follow up should always occur and a review carried out to consider if the medication is still needed and been of benefit in the medical problem or condition.

Student No: 101010101010

Date: 15.12.15

Week No: 3

Prescribing Log No: 1
Client Age: 27   **Sex:** Female

Student Signed ……………………………….

DMP Signed ..………………………………...

Signs and Symptoms (ins PMH, medication, examination, clinical findings, OTC, Allergies)
Post Assessment Diagnosis
Treatment

(Prescribing potential, Dr of NMP) |
| **Drug, name. dose, form, frequency, amount** |
| continue with the daily dosage of one tablet. |

Try to take your pill at about the same time each day.

It may be easiest to take it either last thing at night or first thing in the morning.

Swallow each pill whole, with water if necessary.

I gave her a reminder that the pack is marked with the day of the week on which each pill should be taken

Following the direction of the arrow printed on the pack, you should take one pill each day for 21 days until the strip is empty

Then you have 7 days when you do not take a pill. During the 7 pill-free days, on day 2 or 3, you will have menstruation -like withdrawal bleeding, i.e. your monthly period.

Start your next strip on the 8th day (following the 7 pill free days) – even if the bleeding has not yet ended.

As long as you take Rigevidon correctly, you will always start each new strip on the same day of the week, and you will always have your monthly period on the same day of the month.

If you want to delay your period, you should continue the next pack of Rigevidon, after taking the last pill in the current pack, without a pill-free interval. You can take as many pills from this next pack as you want, until the end of the second blister pack.

When you use the second pack, you may have breakthrough bleeding or spotting. Regular intake of Rigevidon is resumed after the usual 7-day tablet-free interval.

STOP taking Rigevidon immediately and tell your doctor if any of the following symptoms of a blood-clot formation occurs: -

- any unusual, severe or long-lasting headache or migraine

- any sudden changes to your eyesight (such as loss of vision, blurred vision or double vision)

- slurred speech or any other difficulties affecting your speech

- dizziness, fainting or fits

- sudden shortness of breath or difficulty in breathing, sudden coughing for no apparent reason, bloody spittle

- sudden sharp pains in your chest which may reach your left arm

- unusual pain or swelling in your legs

- sudden weakness or numbness in one side or part of your body

- difficulties in moving around (known as motor disturbances)

- severe pain in your abdomen (known as acute abdomen)

Tell your doctor if

- you can feel a lump in your breast.

contra indications - none expected but advised if any adverse reactions to stop and return to surgery.

The Missed Pill Rules: -

What to do if you miss the pill on the first week

Take the most recently missed pill as soon as you remember, even if this means that you have to take 2 tablets at the same time (or in one day). Thereafter, you should continue taking the next pill at the usual time of the day.

You must also use a barrier method of contraception, e.g. a condom, for the next 7 days. If intercourse has taken place during the previous 7 days, the possibility of pregnancy must be considered. The more missed tablets and the closer to the tablet-free interval that this happens, the greater the risk of pregnancy.

What to do if you miss the pill on the second week. Take the most recently missed pill as soon as you remember, even if this means that you have to take 2 tablets at the same time (or in one day). Thereafter, you should continue taking the next pill at the usual time of the day.

Provided the tablets have been taken in a correct manner during the 7 days before the missed tablet, it is not necessary to take further contraceptive measures.

However, if this is not the case, or if more than 1 tablet has been missed, you should take extra contraceptive precautions for 7 days.

What to do if you miss the pill on the third week
The risk of pregnancy is high because of the forthcoming tablet free interval.

The reduced contraceptive protection may, however, be prevented by adjusting the tablet intake. Therefore, by following one of the following two alternatives, it is not necessary to take further contraceptive precautions, provided that all tablets have been taken correctly during the 7 days before the first missed tablet.

If you have not taken Rigevidon correctly during the 7 days before the first missed tablet, you should follow the first of the two alternatives.

Additionally, a barrier method (such as a condom) should be used with the pill for the next 7 days.

Take the most recently missed pill as soon as you remember, even if it means that you have to take 2 tablets at the same time (or in one day). Thereafter, you should continue taking the next pill at the usual time of the day.

You should then start the next pack immediately, i.e. without a tablet-free interval between the packs.

Withdrawal bleeding is unlikely until the end of the second pack, but there may be some spotting, or breakthrough bleeding, on the days you are taking the pill.

2. You may also stop taking tablets from the current pack. In that case, you should keep a period without tablets of up to 7 days, including those days when you forgot to take your tablets, and thereafter continue with the next pack.

If you have missed tablets and then do not get withdrawal bleeding in the first normal tablet-free interval, the possibility of pregnancy must be considered.

The effects of diarrhea and vomiting on the pill. Which are as follows: -

If you have been sick or had diarrhea within 3-4 hours' after taking the pill, your body may not get its usual dose of hormones from that pill. In this case the advice concerning missed pills,
described above should be followed. In case of vomiting or diarrhea, use extra contraceptive precautions, such as a condom, for any intercourse during the stomach upset and for the next 7 days.

I also had a chat with her around sexually transmitted infections so that she can understand the risk of multiple partners, but at present she is in a long-term relationship. Risk of sexually transmitted infections

storage of medicine: -

Do not use Rigevidon after the expiry date which is stated on the package. The expiry date refers to the last day of the month.

This medicinal product does not require any special storage conditions.

Keep out of the reach and sight of children.

Medicines should not be disposed of via wastewater or household

Referral/Review

In 1 months' time

Patient Outcome

(there must be a follow up)

follow up appointment was very straight forward and as expected

She is still taking the COC regular
Her vital signs are all satisfactory
She is still happy with the method
She has no side effects. She asked if she could do a chlamydia test just to make sure all is fine as she has had this previously and she was able to do a self-taken vulvo-vaginal swab under my instruction. The result of this came back as negative.

I was able to tell her no news is good news regarding this and she would hear if it was positive and require a treatment with anti-biotic

Plan to continue with the COC. Return if any side effects or concerns and see a GP.

To have her next review in 2 months and if all okay at this point she may be able to get 6 months' issues at a time

signposted to the local family planning and sexual health clinic if she has any other needs that we cannot meet i.e. wishes for implanon or coil in the future.

Learning Points for Continual Professional Development

This raised the question what is best practice for established pill users and how long should the script be given for.
The DMP and I discussed this and agreed each person should be assessed individually, and that them cannot really be a set straight forward plan in relation to the issue of repeat pills.

Student No: 101010101010

Date: 27.12.15

Week No: 5

Prescribing Log No: 2   **Client Age:**

Sex:

Student Signed …………………………….
DMP Signed ……….………...

Signs and Symptoms (ins PMH, medication, examination, clinical findings, OTC, Allergies)
Post Assessment Diagnosis
Treatment **(Prescribing potential, Dr of NMP)** **Drug, name. dose, form, frequency, amount**
Advice, Referral/Review, Outcome
Lifestyle advice - diet and exercise. Low fat, low carbohydrate diet will encourage weight loss, and also move more -increase activity daily for 20 minutes, increase walking etc. That Desogestrel works by inhibiting ovulation and thickening the cervical mucous. That she will no longer be having the 12 weekly injections. That she can starts the Desogestrel immediately and she must take one tablet every day. Try to take the tablet at the same time each day, either first thing in the morning or at bedtime each day.

This will help to reduce the risk of bleeding also.

That she is covered for contraception as long as she takes the pill each day.

That Depo Provera will still be working so she can assume that although the pill will take 7 days to become effective, the Depo Provera will give her protection during these first 7 days.

The Depo Provera is effective for 14 weeks after having the injection, so we are confident she will be protected during the first 7 days of taking the pill.

When she finishes one packet of pills, she must start the next one immediately.

If you miss taking a pill, or take your pill more than 12 hours late, then you may not be protected against pregnancy.

If you do not start a new strip of pills the following day, then you will not be protected against pregnancy.

The client was also advised about the possibility of irregular bleeding such as:-

Some women will have infrequent bleeding or no periods at all.

Others may experience more frequent or prolonged bleeding that requires sanitary protection.

Over time, bleeding tends to become lighter and less frequent in some women.

That if delayed for 12 hours or more it should be regarded as a missed pill

Barrier method discussed

That taking this pill relies on it been taken at the same time, regularly and every day without a break

She was also advised that is she experiences any side effects to contact the GP surgery immediately and see GP.

Side effects discussed as follows: -

Please return to surgery immediately if you: -

Notice possible signs of a blood clot e.g. severe pain or swelling in either of your legs; unexplained pains in the chest, breathlessness, an unusual cough, especially when you cough up blood (possibly a sign of a thrombosis).

You have a sudden, severe stomach ache or jaundice (you may notice yellowing of the skin, the whites of the eyes, or dark urine, possibly a sign of liver problems).

You feel a lump in your breast (possibly a sign of breast cancer).

You have a sudden or severe pain in the lower abdomen or stomach area (possibly a sign of an ectopic pregnancy - a pregnancy outside the womb).

You are to be immobilized or are to have surgery (consult your doctor at least four weeks in advance).

You have unusual, heavy vaginal bleeding.

You suspect that you are pregnant.

Compliance discussed.

The effects of over the counter medications such as set john's wort discussed.

I also discussed that is she has any
diarrhea and vomiting or disturbances from antibiotics then she will need either to abstain for 7 days or to use alternative contraception, as she may be at risk of pregnancy.

I reminded her to refer to the leaflet in the packet or to contact GP or nurse for advice if concerned or thinks she may be pregnant. That antibiotics can affect the efficacy of the pill.

Referral/Review

In 2 weeks' time

Patient Outcome

Telephone call to client 2 weeks following appointment to review.
Her weight she says is stable.
She is trying to adhere to lifestyle changes

She says she is not very motivated to lose weight.
Encouragement given again today.

She has not had any bleeding yet.

I have advised her some ladies bleed on this method and some do not.

She remains happy with her medication and there are no new concerns noted on review.

Nil side effects noted.

Learning Points for Continual Professional Development

This client was not happy to change method and was persistent in wanting to remain on the Depo Provera. Hence this led me to have a conversation with my DMP around motivation, compliance and concordance in relation to the pill. the discussion to progressed to does the pill ever fail or is failure always due to the user failing to conform to taking it and adhering to the missed pill rules. We won't ever really know - yet I feel it is the motivation of the pill taker that plays the key role in the efficacy of any pill. Refer to Bone Density Scan guidelines and latest Depo Provera Guidance also.

Prescribing Formulary based on specialist areas

This form can be adapted to suit any specific competency area. You may wish to study and gain competence in hypertension or Asthma medications for example, and thus you just adapt.

It is important to discuss this with your designated medical practitioner at the beginning of your course. This will link to your potential prescribing role and will form the basis of your prescribing log, prescriptions and time in practice.

Medication you anticipate prescribing frequently List 20 most common medications (i.e. those you anticipate when qualified you could prescribe on a daily basis/all the time). These medications will reflect your role and qualifications underpinning your specialist area of practice.

Class	Medication	Frequency (daily,	Comments

		weekly)	
Combined Oral Contraceptives (COCs)	Rigevidon oral and most other (COCs)	Daily	
Progestogen Only Pills (POPs)	Desogestrel Oral and most others (POPs)	Daily	
Biguanides	Metformin oral and Metformin Modified Release	Daily	Only Drug in category
Sulphonylureas	Gliclazide Oral and most others	Weekly	In double Therapy
Dipeptidyl peptidase-4 inhibitor (DPP-4 inhibitors)	Sitagliptin and most others		In Triple Therapy

List the medications that you will prescribe infrequently when qualified. These fall within your remit but you anticipate you will not prescribe them as frequently as above.

Class	Medication	Frequency	Comments
Progestegens	Levonorgestrel tablets	Monthly	Emergency Contraception

List the medications which relate to the patients' condition; however, these would not be typical of your potential prescribing practice. If these medications need prescribing this would usually result in referral to a medical prescriber

Class	Medication	Frequency	Comments

Note I am sure that as you go along your journey through Non-Medical Prescribing you may add or change your mind on some medications you first thought you would or would not prescribe.

Once you have stablished your formulary, it is then important to identify your Non-Medical Prescribing lead for your organization and then find your Non-Medical Prescribing Policy for your own specific organization. It is imperative you have one of these policies in place and that if no at no point do you prescribe once qualified until such a policy is in place to give clear guidance on the key issues laid down in the policy example below: -

NON-MEDICAL PRESCRIBING POLICY AND GUIDANCE:

INTRODUCTION

The aim of this policy is to clarify the administrative and procedural steps that are required to enable non-medical prescribers to prescribe safely within your company, hereafter to be referred to as the employer or the company.

SCOPE

This policy applies to non-medical prescribers who are directly employed by the surgery.
Non-medical prescribers can include nurses, midwives, pharmacists, chiropodists/podiatrists, physiotherapists and radiographers with an appropriate prescribing qualification and meeting the requirements of their professional body. Non-medical prescribing at the surgery is anticipated to be by nurse prescribers which is reflected in the policy. However, in the event of other non-medical prescribers such as a pharmacist in direct employment by the surgery, the surgery will amend and update the non-medical prescribing policy.

POLICY STATEMENT

The Surgery will ensure that non-medical prescribing is developed and delivered within the framework of this policy to deliver the National Health Service Agenda for non-medical prescribing:
- to make better use of nurses' skills

- to make it easier for patients to get access to the medicines that they need

DUTIES AND RESPONSIBILITIES

The Surgery's prescribing lead is required to ensure the organization has systems and processes in place to implement this policy.

The Surgery's prescribing lead will ensure that all non-medical prescribers comply with the requirements of this policy and that all prescribing by non-medical prescribers meets the standards required within this policy.

The prescribing lead, if unable to resolve this, should record and submit the reasons on a policy awareness log, discuss this with the non-medical prescriber, prior to a clinical meeting to aim to resolve the issue. This meeting may include, the prescribing lead, executive manager, the non-medical prescriber, a representative from medicines management team and a trade union representative acting on the behalf of the non-medical prescriber. The prescribing lead is responsible for the authorship and the ratification of this policy.

All non-medical prescribers employed by the surgery are required to follow this policy. If this is not possible, the individual should not prescribe and alert their practice manager and prescribing lead by completing an incident form at the earliest point detailing reasons.

PROCEDURES

The surgery's policy on non-medical prescribing is:

Eligibility
Currently to be eligible to prescribe the non-medical prescriber will:
- Be a first level registered nurse or registered pharmacist and all other eligible disciplines

- Have successfully completed a validated Non-Medical Prescribing Training Program

- Has their name annotated on the appropriate professional register?

- Be in a prescribing post

- Have access to a prescribing budget

- Attend regular CPD and strategy group meetings

NURSE INDEPENDENT AND SUPPLEMENTARY PRESCRIBING

Nurse Independent Prescribers are able to prescribe any licensed medicine (i.e. products with a UK marketing authorization) for any medical condition, including some Controlled Drugs. Nurse Independent Prescribers must only prescribe within their own level of experience and competence, acting in accordance with the NMC's 'Code of Professional Conduct: standards for conduct, performance and ethics' (2008).
In line with the NMC (2006) 'Only nurses with relevant knowledge, competence, skills and experience in nursing children should prescribe for children."
A Nurse Independent Prescriber may prescribe an unlicensed medication as an independent nurse prescriber providing:

- You are satisfied an alternative, licensed medication would not meet the

- patient's needs.

- You are satisfied there is a sufficient evidence base and/or experience to demonstrate the medication's safety and efficacy for that particular patient or client.

- You are prepared to take responsibility for prescribing the unlicensed medicine and for overseeing the patient's or client's care, including monitoring and any follow up treatment.

- The patient or client agrees to the prescription in the knowledge that the medicine is unlicensed and understands the implications of this.

- The medication chosen and the reason for choosing it are documented in patient's notes.

- You seek, as necessary, professional advice, for example, from a pharmacist or other authoritative clinical guidance to support your prescribing practice and the specification for the unlicensed medicine.

- You must report suspected adverse drug reactions arising from unlicensed medicines to the Medicines and Healthcare Products Regulatory Agency and CHM via the Yellow Card Scheme. (NMC, 2010, Nurse and midwife independent prescribing of unlicensed medicines.)

The non-medical prescriber is expected to follow best practice guidance for the prescribing of unlicensed medicines by their professional body. Nurse Independent Prescribers may prescribe medicines outside their licensed indications (off-label) where it is accepted clinical practice. In doing so, they are fully accountable and liable for their actions, and should comprehensively document their reasons for prescribing.

Supplementary prescribers may prescribe medicines outside their license if they are included in relevant Clinical Management Plans. Supplementary prescribers are also fully accountable and liable for such prescribing and should comprehensively record their reasons for prescribing.

In all cases of "off-label" prescribing within the surgery, the prescriber is fully accountable and liable for their actions and must be satisfied that:

- An alternative licensed treatment would not meet the patient's needs.

- The prescribed drug and indication is within their area of competence.

- There is satisfactory evidence or experience of safety in prescribing the medication in the circumstances faced.

A Supplementary prescriber would be a nurse who has successfully completed an appropriate validated prescribing training programme and whose name is registered with the relevant professional body with an annotation indicating supplementary prescribing qualification.

Supplementary Prescribing is defined as "a voluntary partnership between an independent prescriber (a doctor or dentist) and a supplementary prescriber (nurse, pharmacist or approved AHP) to implement an agreed patient-specific Clinical Management Plan with the patient's agreement" (Department of Health, 2006), thus enhancing partnership working in a more flexible approach to care delivery (see Appendix 1 – Template for Guidance on Clinical Management Plans and Supplementary Prescribing). Nurse/Pharmacists Independent Prescribers may also utilize supplementary prescribing as part of a clinical management plan (CMP), including unlicensed medications and controlled drugs

PRESCRIPTIONS

Obtaining Prescription Forms

These can be obtained after University, NMC and Health Authority requirements have been meet from: Dispatch Office.

Prescription Pad Security

The Surgery will maintain a list of signatories of all prescribers who prescribe for patients who are directly employed by the surgery. All prescribers must provide a specimen signature to the Health Authority. Prescription pads are the property of the Surgery. It is the responsibility of the prescriber to ensure security of the prescription pad always.

Prescribers should keep a record of the serial numbers of the prescriptions in the pad issued to them. The prescriber and employing organization should record the first and last serial number of the prescription pad.

It is also good practice for prescribers to record the number of the first and last remaining forms of an in-use pad at the end of a day on which it is used, this should be recorded in a place separate from the prescription pad. If a prescription pad is unused for four weeks, the first and last serial number needs to be checked.

The prescription pad should only be produced when needed and never left unattended.
The prescription pad must not be left on the desk but placed in a locked drawer, locked filing cabinet or locked cupboard.

Under no circumstances should blank prescription forms be signed before use.
When travelling between patients the prescription pad must not be visible and ideally kept in a bag with a combination lock.

Loss of Prescription Forms

It is anticipated that electronic generated will be used primarily, however, in the event of a printer failure or home visits hand generated prescriptions may require. In the event of prescriptions ordered but not received, the Dispatch Office and practice manager must be notified and they will make appropriate enquiries.

Prescribers should report the loss or theft of prescription forms to their Practice manager and to add here as soon as the loss/theft is discovered. The following information will be required:

- Prescribers name

- Professional registration number (NMC number)

- First and last serial numbers of prescription forms

- Details of loss/theft.

The executive manager must ensure that the loss/theft has been reported and that an incident form is completed by the prescriber.

On termination of employment prescribers must ensure that their prescription forms are returned to the dispatch office.

RECORD KEEPING

All prescribers are required to keep contemporaneous records, which are unambiguous, legible and in accordance with the of the prescriber's professional body.
A record of a prescription should be entered the patient's notes (as appropriate) at time of writing or at the shortest possible interval thereafter.

The time between writing a prescription and recording in the clinical records should not normally exceed 48 hours from writing the prescription. (To take account of Bank Holidays).

The record should include:

- Date

- Name of prescriber

- Name of item prescribed

- Form

- Dose duration/quantity to be dispensed and frequency

- Quantity and treatment duration

- Advice given on over the counter items

- Advice on any treatments to be discontinued or adjusted

- Summary of presentation

- Rational for prescribing

- Record of any allergies

- If in the judgement of the prescriber it is necessary to advise the patient's doctor immediately of a prescription, this action should be recorded in the patient records.

If Supplementary Prescribing is undertaken, a Clinical Management Plan (CMP) is completed (in appendix) scanned in the patient's communications and the original copy kept in the paper records.

ADVERSE DRUG REACTION (ADR) REPORTING

It is the responsibility of all healthcare professionals to report all ADRs and not just the prescriber. The prescriber should report adverse drug reactions for all black triangle drugs, herbal medicines, those occurring in patients under 18 or not a known or predicted reaction. Reporting must be to the Medicines and Healthcare Products Regulatory Agency (MHRA)/Commission on Human Medicines by use of the Yellow Card Adverse Drug Reactions Reporting Scheme.

If a patient suffers a suspected adverse reaction to a prescribed, over the counter or herbal medicine it must be reported to the prescriber.

Yellow cards are found at the back of the BNF or can be completed online (www.yellowcard.gov.uk). Only serious adverse reactions for established drugs, but all suspected adverse reactions for black triangle drugs, should be reported.

Details of any adverse reaction and any action taken must be clearly and comprehensively documented in the patient's clinical notes. (see record keeping above).

GOOD PRACTICE, ETHICS AND ISSUES COMMON TO ALL PRESCRIBERS

In the event of an adverse incident or a near miss, prescribers must adhere to the surgery policy for the reporting and management of adverse incidents.
The prescriber is accountable for all his/her prescribing decisions.
The prescriber should only prescribe for a patient whom she/he has assessed for care, on an approved prescription form. Non-medical prescribers must work within their competency and ensure patients are aware of the scope and limitations of non-medical prescribing.

Prescribers should not prescribe for themselves, close family or friends because objectivity or judgement may be impaired and clinical examinations impossible.

Any prescriber who writes and signs a prescription assumes full responsibility and clinical liability for it (the surgery will accept vicarious liability for employees working within the framework of this policy).

Repeat prescribing

The non-medical prescriber may issue repeat prescriptions within their competencies and boundaries of own formulary, following face to face assessment of the patient.

The non-medical prescriber should review a repeat prescription following a maximum of 6 prescriptions or 6 months, whichever is reached first.
Suitable monitoring for each patient's condition should be in place to ensure those requiring further assessment do not receive repeat prescriptions without being seen by an appropriate prescriber.

Pharmaceutical Company Representatives

Please refer to the surgery's policy for Pharmaceutical industry and gifts policy.

Legal and Clinical Liability

Where a prescriber is appropriately trained and qualified and prescribes as part of their professional duties with the consent of the employer, the employer is held vicariously liable for their actions. In addition, prescribers are individually professionally accountable to their professional body for this aspect of their practice and must at all times act in accordance with their relevant Code of Professional Conduct.

It is the surgery's responsibility to provide professional indemnity insurance. All prescribers should ensure that professional indemnity insurance cover is in place for a prescribing role.

Verification of Prescribing Status

Most queries will generally be from pharmacists and will be resolved by telephoning the prescriber or the prescriber's employer. The surgery will maintain a list of signatories of all prescribers.

General queries about the qualification of a prescriber can be made by via the internet **http://www.nmc-uk.org/**

SUPERVISION STATEMENT

The Department of Health (2006) recommends that nurse independent prescribers should use clinical supervision arrangements as an opportunity for reflection on prescribing and other aspects of practice. "clinical supervision is regular, protected time for facilitated, in-depth reflection on clinical practice. It aims to enable the supervisee to achieve, sustain and creatively develop a high quality of practice through means of focus, support and development." (Bond 1998).

The employer has a responsibility to ensure prescribers have access to undertake relevant clinical supervision and CPD as identified through individual appraisals. This should include regular ongoing clinical supervision with an independent prescriber/GP PACT data should be discussed quarterly initially with the non-medical prescriber as part of regular clinical supervision.

The non-medical prescriber is responsible for accessing regular clinical supervision regarding prescribing practice as provided by the employer.

NMC recommends that appraisal of CPD needs for prescribing should be undertaken annually as part of performance review (2008). During this review issues around expanding the non-medical prescriber's formulary and competence to do so should be addressed and confirmed/declined. It is the responsibility of the non-medical prescriber to access relevant education and training to keep up to date with clinical and professional developments and maintain their competence in prescribing.

Continuing Professional Development needs to meet requirements for competence for the prescribers' safe practice and their professional governing body.

EQUALITY AND DIVERSITY

Prescribers will ensure that those with barriers to communication and reduced
capacity is provided with additional support to enable them to exercise the same
informed decisions as those without such barriers.

MENTAL CAPACITY

Non-medical prescribers should be aware of the principles of the Mental Capacity Act when prescribing medication, and providing information to help individuals make informed choices about medication including non-pharmacological options:

- A presumption of capacity - every adult has the right to make his or her own decisions and must be assumed to have capacity to do so unless it is proved otherwise;

- The right for individuals to be supported to make their own decisions – people must be given all appropriate help before anyone concludes that they cannot make their own decisions;

- That individuals must retain the right to make what might be seen as eccentric or unwise decisions;

- Best interests – anything done for or on behalf of people without capacity must be in their best interests; and

- Least restrictive intervention – anything done for or on behalf of people without capacity should be the least restrictive of their basic rights and freedoms.

IMPLEMENTATION

The implementation of this policy requires continued commitment from executive manager and prescribing lead to allow sufficient time and economic investment in continued professional development activities for the individual non-medical prescriber. In order to maintain prescribing competency, the surgery must allow non-medical prescribers sufficient opportunity to prescribe on a regular basis.

MONITORING AND AUDIT

All prescribing in the surgery is monitored and audited on a regular basis by the prescribing lead, executive manager, self-auditing and by the externally by a medicines management pharmacist. Non-medical prescribers will additionally be audited when other prescribing audits are identified in the surgery.

Nurse Independent and Supplementary Prescribing Assessment Competencies

The assessment varies from organization to organization however there are key competencies which must be achieved and demonstrated within learning logs. We have already looked at prescribing logs and examples previously. Now let us consider learning logs and their relation to the competency framework.

Single competency framework for all prescribers (May 2012)

Prescribing competencies in relation to teaching, learning & assessment (National Prescribing Centre 2012) *The course will also enable you to be a supplementary prescriber therefore these should also still be achieved (see separate prescribing ompetencies)*

The prescribing Competency framework
Domain A: The consultation

Competency 1: Knowledge
Has up-to-date clinical, pharmacological and pharmaceutical knowledge relevant to own area of practice.

1. Understands the conditions being treated, their natural progress and how to assess their severity.

2. Understands different non-pharmacological and pharmacological approaches to modifying disease and promoting health, identifies and assesses the desirable outcomes of treatment.

3. Understands the mode of action and pharmacokinetics of medicines and how these mechanisms may

be altered (e.g. by age, renal impairment), and how this affects treatment decisions.

4. Understands the potential for adverse effects and how to avoid/minimise, recognise and manage them.

5. Uses up-to-date information about relevant products (e.g. formulations, pack sizes, storage conditions, costs).

6. Applies the principles of evidence-based practice, including clinical and cost-effectiveness.

7. Aware of how medicines are licensed, sourced and supplied, and the implications for own prescribing.

8. Knows how to detect and report suspected adverse drug reactions.

9. Understands the public health issues related to medicines and their use.

10. Appreciates the potential for misuse of medicines.

11. Understands antimicrobial resistance and the roles of infection prevention, control and antimicrobial stewardship measures as outlined in the ARHAI and PHE Antimicrobial Prescribing and Stewardship Competences

Competency 2: Options

Makes or reviews a diagnosis, generates management options for the patient and follows up management.

12. Takes an appropriate medical history and medication history which includes both current and previously
prescribed and non-prescribed medicines, supplements and complementary remedies, and allergies and intolerances.

13. Undertakes an appropriate clinical assessment using relevant equipment and techniques.

14. Accesses and interprets relevant patient records to ensure knowledge of the patient's management.

15. Makes, or understands, the working or final diagnosis by considering and systematically deciding between the various possibilities (differential diagnosis).

16. Requests and interprets relevant investigations.

17. Considers all treatment options including no treatment, non-pharmacological interventions and medicines
usage.

18. Assesses the effect of multiple pathologies, existing medication, allergies and contraindications on management options.

19. Assesses the risks and benefits to the patient of taking or, not taking a medicine or treatment.

20. Where a medicine is appropriate, identifies the different options.

21. Establishes and maintains a plan for reviewing the therapeutic objective, discharge or end point of treatment.

22. Ensures that the effectiveness of treatment and potential unwanted effects are monitored.

23. Makes changes to the treatment plan in light of on-going monitoring and the patient's condition and preferences.

24. Communicates information about medicines and what they are being used for when sharing or transferring prescribing responsibilities/information.

Competency 3: Shared decision making
(with parents, care-givers or advocates where appropriate) Establishes a relationship based on trust and mutual respect. Recognises patients as partners in the consultation.

25. Identifies and respects the patient's values, beliefs and expectations about medicines.

26. Takes into account the nature of peoples' diversity when prescribing.

27. Undertakes the consultation in an appropriate setting taking account of confidentially, dignity and respect.

28. Adapts consultations to meet needs of different patients (e.g. for language, age, capacity, physical or sensory impairments).

29. Deals sensitively with patients' emotions and concerns about their medicines.

30. Creates a relationship which does not encourage the expectation that a prescription will be supplied.

31. Explains the rationale behind and the potential risks and benefits of management options.

32. Works with patients to make informed choices about their management and respects their right to refuse or limit treatment.

33. Aims for an outcome of the consultation with which the patient and prescriber are satisfied.

34. When possible, supports patients to take responsibility for their medicines and self-manage their conditions.

35. Gives the patient clear accessible information about their medicines (e.g. what it is for, how to use it, where to get it from, possible unwanted effects).

36. Checks patient's understanding of and commitment to their management, monitoring and follow-up.

37. Understands the different reasons for non-adherence to medicines (practical and behavioural) and how best to support patients. Routinely assesses adherence in a non-judgemental way.

Domain B: Prescribing Effectively

GOOD PRESCRIBING

Competency 4: Safe
Is aware of own limitations. Does not compromise patient safety.

38. Knows the limits of their own knowledge and skill, and works within them.

39. Knows when to refer to or seek guidance from another member of the team or a specialist.

40. Only prescribes a medicine with adequate, up-to-date awareness of its actions, indications, dose, contraindications, interactions, cautions, and side effects (using, for example, the BNF/BNFC).

41. Accurately calculates doses and routinely checks calculations where relevant, for example for children.

42. Keeps up to date with advances in practice and emerging safety concerns related to prescribing.

43. Knows about common types of medication errors and how to prevent them.

44. Ensures confidence and competence to prescribe are maintained.

45. Makes accurate, legible and contemporaneous records and clinical notes of prescribing decisions.

46. Effectively uses the systems necessary to prescribe medicines (e.g. medicine charts, electronic prescribing, decision support).

47. Writes legible, unambiguous and complete prescriptions which meet legal requirements.

Competency 5: Professional
Ensures prescribing practice is consistent with scope of practice, organisational, professional and regulatory standards, guidance and codes of conduct.

48. Accepts personal responsibility for prescribing and understands the legal and ethical implications of doing so.

49. Makes prescribing decisions based on the needs of patients and not the prescriber's personal considerations.

50. Knows and applies legal and ethical frameworks affecting prescribing practice (e.g. misuse of drugs regulations, prescribing of unlicensed/off label medicines).

51. Takes responsibility for own learning and continuing professional development.

52. Maintains patient confidentiality in line with best practice and regulatory standards and contractual requirements.

Competency 6: Always improving
Actively participates in the review and development of prescribing practice to optimise patient outcomes.

53. Learns and changes from reflecting on practice.

54. Shares and debates own and others prescribing practice, and acts upon feedback and discussion.

55. Acts upon colleagues' inappropriate prescribing practice using appropriate mechanisms.

56. Understands and uses tools to improve prescribing (e.g. review of prescribing data, audit and feedback).

57. Reports prescribing errors and near misses, reviews practice to prevent recurrence.

58. Makes use of networks for support, reflection and learning

Domain C: Prescribing in context

Competency 7: The healthcare system
Understands and works within local and national policies, processes and systems that impact on prescribing practice. Sees how own prescribing impacts on the wider healthcare community.

59. Understands and works within local frameworks for medicines use as appropriate (e.g. local formularies, care pathways, protocols and guidelines).

60. Understands the need to work with, or develop, safe systems and processes locally to support prescribing, for example, repeat prescribing, transfer of information about medicines.

61. Works within the NHS/organisational or other ethical code of conduct when dealing with the pharmaceutical industry.

62. Understands budgetary constraints and prioritisation processes at local and national level (health-care resources are finite).

63. Understands the national frameworks for medicines use (e.g. *NICE, SMC, AWMSG and medicines management/optimisation).

64. Prescribes generically where appropriate, practical and safe for the patient.

Competency 8: Information
Knows how to access relevant information. Can use and apply information in practice

65. Understands the advantages and limitations of different information sources available to prescribers.

66. Accesses relevant, up-to-date information using trusted evidence-based resources.

67. Regularly reviews the evidence base behind therapeutic strategies.

Competency 9: Self and others
Works in partnership with colleagues for the benefit of patients. Is self-aware and confident in own ability as a prescriber.

68. Thinks and acts as part of a multidisciplinary team to ensure that continuity of care is developed and not compromised.

69. Establishes relationships with other professionals based on understanding, trust and respect for each other's roles in relation to prescribing.

70. Recognises and deals with pressures that might result in inappropriate prescribing (for example, pharmaceutical industry, media, patient, colleagues).

71. Negotiates the appropriate level of support and supervision for role as a prescriber.

72. Provides support and advice to other prescribers where appropriate.

Glossary — Non-medical prescribing

Non-medical prescribing
Non-medical prescribing is prescribing by specially trained nurses, optometrists, pharmacists, physiotherapists, podiatrists and radiographers, working within their clinical competence as either independent and/or supplementary prescribers.

Independent prescribing
Independent prescribing is prescribing by a practitioner, who is responsible and accountable for the assessment of patients with undiagnosed or diagnosed conditions and for decisions about the clinical management required, including prescribing. In practice, there are TWO distinct forms of non-medical independent prescriber.

i) An independent prescriber may currently be a specially trained nurse, pharmacist or optometrist who can prescribe any licensed medicine within their clinical competence. Nurse and pharmacist independent prescribers can also prescribe unlicensed medicines and controlled drugs.

ii) A community practitioner nurse prescriber (CPNP), for example district nurse, health visitor or school nurse, can independently prescribe from a limited formulary called the Nurse Prescribers' Formulary for

Competency	Statement
Domain A: The Consultation	
A	Reviews diagnosis and generates management options for the patient within the clinical management plan.

Community Practitioners, which can be found in the British National Formulary (BNF).

Supplementary prescribing

Supplementary prescribing is a voluntary partnership between a doctor or dentist and a supplementary prescriber to prescribe within an agreed patient-specific clinical management plan (CMP) with the patient's agreement.

Nurses, optometrists, pharmacists, physiotherapists, podiatrists and radiographers may currently train as supplementary prescribers and once qualified may prescribe any medicine within their clinical competence, according to the CMP.

The regulators of non-medical prescribers
Professional regulators are required to set standards of education, training, conduct and performance and approve education programmes that prepare healthcare professionals to prescribe. They record the qualification of prescriber on their register. The regulators are:
Nursing and Midwifery Council (for nurses and midwives)

General Pharmaceutical Council (for pharmacists)

General Optical Council (for optometrists)

Health Professions Council (for physiotherapists, podiatrists and radiographers)

	Always follows up management.
B	Reviews medical history and medication history which includes both current and previously prescribed and non-prescribed medicines, supplements and complimentary remedies, and allergies and intolerances.
C	Reviews the clinical condition using relevant equipment and techniques.
D	Reviews the working or final diagnosis.
E	Where a medicine is appropriate, identifies the different options in the clinical management plan.
F	Makes changes within the clinical management plan in light of ongoing monitoring and the patient's condition and preferences.
Domain B: Prescribing Effectively	
G	Knows how and when to refer back to, or seek guidance from, the independent prescriber, another member of the team or a specialist.
H	Understand the scope of own prescribing responsibility in the context of a shared clinical management plan.
I	Ensures that the patient consents to be managed by a prescribing partnership.
Domain C: Prescribing in Context	
J	Understands the principles behind supplementary prescribing and how they are applied in practice.
K	Proactively negotiates with the independent prescriber to develop clinical management plans.

NON-MEDICAL PRESCRIBING MODULE
LEARNING LOG TEMPLATE EXAMPLES

STUDENT NO:

Date: 12.11.2015

MODULE No:

Session duration: 2 Hrs

DMP present YES/N0

DMP HRS =

TOTAL HOURS =

Student signed: _____

DMP Signed: _____

LEARNING LOG

Venue – i.e. Clinic. GP surgery, Patient home, meeting

DMP present – yes or no

RELEVANT COMPETENCE AND TOPIC

59. Understands and works within local frameworks for medicines use as appropriate (e.g. local formularies, care pathways, protocols and guidelines.

64. Prescribes generically where appropriate, practical and safe for the patient

66. Accesses relevant, up-to-date information using trusted evidence-based resources.

EVIDENCE OF ACHIEVEMENT OF COMPETENCY

I arranged a visit with the local CCG pharmacist.

This enabled me to learn about the local frameworks for medicines management. I learned how to access the CCG pharmacy guidelines online. I must adhere to when considering. I explored algorithms on medication for treatment of diabetes type II. I discussed red/amber/green drug lists and the significance of the same. I learned about antibiotic stewardship. I can take vigilance back to practice from this. I could now signpost other professionals to this site.

I found clear evidence to prescribe generically within these formularies and algorithms. I found that this has taught me that there is really a flow chart or guidance on everything I could think of in practice. I found a wealth of practical, safe, well researched evidence that I can utilise in practice when I am a qualified NMP. I also learned that it may be possible to bring some of these to protected time for learning, to ensure that I am supporting my prescribing colleagues, and assisting them in their decision making and updates also. I also learned that this would be a good way to continue to professionally develop once I have qualified as a NMP. The impact of this on my role as a newly qualified NMP, will be that I have up to date evidence based prescribing guidelines available ready for access online.

NON-MEDICAL PRESCRIBING MOD.ULE LEARNING LOG TEMPLATE EXAMPLE

STUDENT NO:

Date:

MODULE No:

Session duration: 3 Hrs

DMP present YES/N0
DMP HRS =

TOTAL HOURS =

Student signed: _____
DMP Signed: _____

LEARNING LOG

Venue – i.e. Clinic. GP surgery, Patient home, meeting
DMP present – yes or no

RELEVANT COMPETENCE AND TOPIC

24. Communicates information about medicines and what they are been used for when sharing or transferring prescribing responsibilities and information.

31. Explains the rationale and potential risks and benefits of management options.

EVIDENCE OF ACHIEVEMENT OF COMPETENCY

Today I had a discussion with my DMP around who has prescribing rights. I identified areas of concern where clients going into secondary care, palliative care or residential and nursing home care also. I learned that there the communication between GP practices, secondary care and the community care homes have a great deal of room for development and that it is not streamlined as it ought to be. I learned that it is vital to access the capacity of everyone in practice, before prescribing drugs, as mental capacity can impact on the ability to ensure medication safety when prescribing. I learned that is vital to ensure the risks of prescribing verses the risks of not especially with clients with a risk of dementia, early dementia and ongoing or acute dementia also. I learned that we have just had some input with a GP - who has been allocated to our surgery to asset in the diagnosis of dementia and to review all dementia medications also. I learned to acknowledge my limitations with prescribing for dementia clients and to use resources available and refer when in doubt and not prescribe without bearing all these facts in mind when qualified as a NMP I learned also that there are tools to help assess capacity of system one and via the NHS I also learned that it is suggested that prescribing responsibilities should not be split.

I considered and learnt what prescribing responsibilities meant and recognised that I had not understood this previously. I learned that to identify who has responsibility for prescribing of all medicines I would need to refer to the HERPC red and amber drug alerts to establish who has responsibility. I reviewed some other organisations red, amber and green drug alerts for comparison and as a learning exercise. I learnt that there is strict guidance on transferring prescribing care to secondary care, palliative care and to refer to guidance for healthcare professionals in the Hull and East Riding Area. I learnt that for further advice I could contact the relevant Pharmaceutical Advisor., or specialist. However, this means to me within practice that I need to be aware that this system is in place, but this would be an area when I can clearly identify my limitations within my scope of practice as a NMP and I would refer to GP and not act here. Transfer of Care and prescribing rights is beyond my scope and shall continue to be once

> I qualify as a NMP, never the less I shall be vigilant with these thoughts whilst in practice. I learned that there is other guidance on the transferring of prescribing available from the GMC also. I learnt that there is guidance from the NHS England on red, amber and green medication status I learned that NICE medicines practice guidelines provide recommendations for good practice for those individuals and organisations involved in governing, commissioning, prescribing and decision-making about medicines. I recognised the importance of been aware of the NICE guidance

Following completion of each log a reference list must be maintained as evidence as to where information this accessed. These learning logs can also count against re-validation. Dependent on where you are studying you Non-Medical Prescribing you will sit different theory and practical assignments. If you are required to maintain and submit a portfolio both the prescribing logs and learning logs will need to be submitted as evidence of achievement of both practical and theory. It is a nice professional approach to start your portfolio with an introduction as to the Journey you are about to embark on. An example of my own introduction follows.

Introduction

Having qualified as a Registered Genera Nurse over 20 years ago, I have a strong professional career that spans over both the acute and primary care sectors. The journey took me into the community in 2003, when I completed my BSc Hons Community Specialist Practitioner qualification, combined with the V100 Community Practice Nurse Prescribing course. This allowed nurses to a limited access of medicines.

During the past few years I have been working in Practice Nursing and thus have been working mostly with long term conditions. Having completed the Diabetes Diploma, it is evident that I have much knowledge and skills to consult with diabetic patients to assess them needs, review their care and to plan care to maximize their health. Furthermore, I progressed to complete the Sexual Health and Family Planning courses and once again had the liberty of consulting with these patients daily. I work daily completing pill checks and using Patient Group Directives for contraception such as Depo Provera.

As my career progressed within the two areas above such as diabetes and contraception advice, it has become apparent that it would be beneficial to the client's if I could prescribe within these two areas, where I practice routinely daily. The gap in training and qualifications became apparent in relation to these two areas, which identified to me the present area for study within the Non-Medical Prescribing module.

Having considered my professional scope of practice, and a desire to work more holistically, I made the conscious decision to study the Non-Medical Prescribing Module. Thus, this introduction will set the scene for a journey of competency based assessment and professional development into the realms of Non-Medical Prescribing. Waite and Keenan (2010) highlighted the importance of competency based assessment as a means of continued professional development. It is anticipated that my competency and knowledge and decision making process will develop me to a consciously competent practitioner. I hope to enhance my knowledge into specific drugs such as oral contraceptives and sulfonylurea's. I anticipate that I will have the opportunity to develop my awareness in relation to these specific drugs and the interactions and contra-indications of these drugs also. I will also consider and re-visit anatomy and physiology and consider pharmacology in great depth.

This process will hopefully identify areas and opportunities for learning and enable me to fulfil the transition into Non-Medical Prescribing. I anticipate that I will have the opportunity to consultant with many clients who have a diabetes. I hope to gain great support from my Designated Medical Practitioner and many other professional colleagues. I acknowledge that my knowledge is limited in pharmacology, drug legislation, contra-indications and the side effects of drugs also. I acknowledge that my consultation method may be based more on a nursing model rather that a medical model and hope to consider this in detail. Orem (1995) discussed the self-care model of nursing. This is the approach I feel I encourage within practice today. However, Neighbour (2005) a model which looks at the consultation in a different light. This seems to indicate that looking at our self during the consultation, and questioning our approach may be the best approach. Indicating that we may need to adapt each consultation. I will seek feedback from clients on the consultation to identify if I can adapt my approach or if it seems to meet the need of the client in the manner I performed it.

I will explore prescribing in practice in relation to a small formulary of drugs which I have clearly identified as Sulfonylurea drugs and oral contraceptives. I feel I can demonstrate the underpinning knowledge of diabetes and contraception with the qualification I hold in these area of practice, but would like to develop this level of competence also. It is important to highlight, that I will not be prescribing for children under the age of 16.

This I hope sets out my experience, background and history within health care and the qualifications I have obtained. I shall be reflecting on this and using this to enable me to develop myself towards the role of Non-Medical Prescriber. During the journey, I shall log learning objectives, plans and outcomes to identify what I may have done well, what I may do differently, what I have learnt, what I have achieved, would I prescribe if qualified and if so what would I prescribe and why. I will follow up clients to assess and review whether they suffered any side effects of medications and to gain their feedback on their experience and our consultation.

I envisage that the impact of the above will all impact on practice in many ways. It will allow me to work more holistically, opportunistically and to play a bigger part in the team. I hope to enhance the clients experience and make their care timelier and to use new competencies to meet patient requirements.

There will also be some assignment requirements for submission at either level 6 or 7 study.

Please see sample assignments on The Consultation and Reflection (OSCE).

The Consultation Essay

Is Desogestrel as effective as a combined oral contraception?

I currently work as a practice nurse, in general practice and assist with contraception choices. My formulary focuses on both combined oral contraceptives (COCs) and progestogen only pills (POPs). Brand Cerazette POP is available now in its active ingredient form of Desogestrel (DSG), which can be described as a 3rd generation 19-

nortestosterone derivative progestogen. (Grandi et al, 2014). Both COCs and POPs are safe, effective choices for contraception (National Institute for Health and Care Excellence (NICE, 2015; British National Formulary (BNF), 2015-2016).

Desogestrel is a prescription only medication and its indication for use in as oral POP, in females of childbearing age. The dosage is one tablet (75mcg each) daily and it is safe in pregnancy, does not affect lactation, contra-indicated in porphyria, caution must be applied in liver disease and it can increase the risk of breast cancer (BNF, 2015-2016) Presently there are no concerns regarding the safety of DSG and no black triangle warning with the drug.

Currently the pharmacological treatment options for using DSG are COC or POP. DSG is contained in many oral contraceptive presentations (Grandi et al 2014; BNF 2015-2016). DSG is contained in some COCs to ethinyl-estradiol (EE) or alone in a POP. Its principal metabolite (etonogestrel, ETN) is the only progestin used for intravaginal combined contraception and one of the most used for subdermal hormonal contraception (Grandi et al, 2014). When used as a POP, it is believed to be highly effective and as efficient as COC (Korver et al, 2005), and it is available on the National Health Service (NHS).

When considering prescribing DSG, it is vital to understand and determine what cause may have what effect as discussed by (Lawman and Browne, 2005), with the outcome aimed to do well and not cause harm. Understanding the evidence that DSG used as a POP is safe and effective and is a better choice rather than a COC is vital, when considering prescribing.

We know that COC comes with a risk of thromboembolism (Sidney et al, 2012), (BNF, 2015), whereas DSG comes with no risk (Benagiano and Primiero, 2003). (The summary of product characteristics for (SPC), Desogestrel, 2015) indicate that the pharmacokinetics of oral dosing of DSG are firstly rapid absorption and conversion into etonogestrel (ENG). If there are normal steady-state conditions, then the peak serum levels are reached 1.8 hours after taking the tablet and the absolute bioavailability of ENG is approximately 70% at this point. The body will then distribute the ENG which is 95.5-99% bound to serum proteins, predominantly to albumin and sex hormone binding globulin but on a lower extent. For metabolism to occur the DSG goes through the process of hydroxylation and dehydrogenation and is converted into the active metabolite ENG and metabolized via sulphate and glucuronide conjugation. Elimination of the drug occurs with a mean half-life of approximately 30 hours. The (SPC, 2015) state there is no difference with single or multiple dosing, and that steady-state levels in plasma are reached after 4-5 days. Excretion occurs via the faces, urine and in breast milk.

The pharmacodynamics of this drug are that primarily it inhibits ovulation (Korver et al, 2005; BNF, 2016), and secondly it thickens the cervical mucus. It has been established (Korver et al, 2005; Benagino and Primiero, 2003) that with DSG ovulation is inhibited for up to 36 hours and it has a missed pill window of 12 hours. This is believed due to the active ingredient DSGs ability to inhibit the production and circulation of progesterone circulating levels and its impact on inhibiting follicular growth during menstrual cycles. In practice this means the mode of action offers greater reliability and flexibility than other POP. Other POPs do not inhibit ovulation and are only effective for up to 27 hours, giving them a 3-hour 'missed pill' window.

(Rice et al, 1999) carried out a study based on the inhibition of ovulation achieved by DSG and found only 1:103 women would ovulate, giving a 95% confidence in the efficacy. If taking the tablet is delayed for 12 hours or more it is regarded as a missed pill (BNF, 2015-2016), perhaps this is the reason the 1:103 women ovulate?

After a review of the evidence I found no evidence to confirm any other POP inhibits ovulation. (Rice et al, 1999; Korver et al, 2005) suggest that the pearl index of woman using DSG is comparable to COCs, meaning that it is as effective as a COC, and safer due to a lower risk of venous embolus. Recent evidence however (Ziller et al, 2014; MHRA 2014), suggests the risk of a venous embolus in any women taking a COC is low. A study by (Stegeman et al, 2013) found that both the choice of progestogen used and the dose of ethinylestradiol, were key to reducing the risk.

This knowledge will inform and evidence practice that DSG has proven efficacy, when
taken regularly as prescribed. (Baxter, 2010), identified common interactions with DSG such as Orlistat, Lamotrigine, St. Johns' Wort and anti-epileptics. Orlistat can induce severe diarrhoea and this will reduce the bioavailability of the drug (Baxter, 2010). DSG might increase lamotrigine levels and adverse effects (Baxter 2010), and therefore caution

should be applied on patients taking this drug. St Johns' wort will reduce the efficacy of oral contraceptives (Hall et al, 2003; Zhou et al, 2004). St Johns' Wort is an inducer of cytochrome P450 family 3A enzymes and these reduce the efficacy of oral contraceptives. Caution should also be applied in women using anti-epileptics Baxter, 2010).

Overall, the available evidence suggests DSG is a safe and effective contraception (NICE, 2015). There is no evidence to support the use of DSG in the under 18s or for patients with renal and hepatic impairment. DSG does inhibit ovulation (Korver et al, 2005; Benagino and Primiero, 2003; Rice et al, 1999). It is as effective as a COC (Korver et al, 2005; Benagino and Primiero, 2003; Rice et al, 1999), with a pearl index equal to a COC, when taken regularly. It is a good choice of POP as it is cheap, can be prescribed generically and is available in good supply within the NHS. The ongoing outcome can be cheaply and easily monitored within practice. There are minimal interactions to note and no safety concerns with (DSG). Having considered all the above and the knowledge I acquired about this drug, I would prescribe it when qualified.

Assignment Reflection (OSCE)
Reflective Account of Objective Structured Clinical Examination (OSCE)

My Designated Medical Prescriber (DMP) chose a patient at random, booked in for a contraceptive pill check for purpose of my observed structured clinical examination (OSCE). The purpose of this is to test the practical skills, attitudes and knowledge and is a form of exam (Wolfgang et al, 2013). The skills of the DMP are imperative in the process and (Hurley et al, 2015) suggest that the reliability and accuracy of the inter observer can vary between 73 - 93% and this identifies that it is also, important to obtain feedback from the client also.

As a Practice Nurse my role in the OSCE was to assess, gather information, plan and implement appropriate care. I did so utilising evidence based guidance such as the (Faculty of Sexual Health and

Reproductive Health, UKMEC, 2016), Contraception – progestogen-only methods (National Institute for Health and Care Excellence (NICE), 2015) and British National Formulary, BNF 70, 2015-2016).

For this reflective account, I utilized a reflective cycle by Gibbs, (1988) as I find this a simple but effective reflection tool. I decided to use the Calgary Cambridge Consultation Model (Silverman et al, 2013), because it provides a structure in 5 key areas to support building the relationship.

To set the scene the OSCE was carried out within General Practice in a nurse led clinic and observed by my DMP. Whilst initiating the session I identified that the client was female and aged 36 years old. I had never consulted with this lady before and thus had no prior knowledge to draw from but this was not a problem and I felt comfortable.

To gather information prior to the consultation I accessed her records on Systmone (S1) and I identified that she was an established pill user and S1 enabled me to gather information before the client enters the room. In doing so I established that she was taking Desogestrel 75mcg one tablet daily and could recognise that I am familiar with this drug. I felt comfortable and relaxed in my knowledge.

At this stage of the consultation I was anticipating that I would use my knowledge of guidelines such as Contraception - progestogen-only methods (NICE, 2015). I was also, mindful to have the (British National Formulary (BNF 70,

2015-16) available for review during the consultation.

Whilst initiating the session I felt confident that I was working within my sphere of competence, because I am qualified within contraception and pill checks are routine practice. I set about and performed a sequence of events for gathering information, physical examination and anticipated these would inform my clinical decision and evidence base for decision making.

After welcoming the patient in and introducing myself, I obtained consent and this is important to identify that I have gained simple open permission during the clinical decision making process. Consent was necessary to ensure I am acting with accountability and adhering to the (Nursing and Midwifery Council (NMC), The Code for nurses and midwives 2015), not only for the consultation but also for the purpose of the OSCE and the presence of my DMP.

Within practice my priority was patient safety and to maintain this I confirmed her name, date of birth and age to ensure her safety. This is vital to prevent omissions and errors and this will safeguard the client (Silverman et al, 2013). The benefit of
this is that I am then assured I am utilizing the correct clinical record, and thus I am reviewing the correct medical information again ensuring her safety.

(The Code, NMC, 2015) recommend safety and accurate record keeping and stress the importance of vigilance when utilizing the same. This ensures a clinical history is maintained within the client's medical records.

I confirmed the purpose of the appointment was a POP contraception review. I confirmed that the lady wished to remain on this method and she stressed clearly absolutely she did, as she is in a relationship and requires contraception. The consultation progressed with a physical assessment and gathering of base line data such as blood pressure 139/77, heart rate 87 and these are within the normal range.

Her body mass index (BMI) 33 plus and this is raised and a (UKMEC, 2016) category1 consideration, but this is deemed safe when using a POP. She is an ex-smoker and drinks minimal alcohol so no further health promotion was required, other than drawing her attention to her BMI.

Gathering of such data is vital to identify what her base line measurements are to ensure I obtain a clear picture of her general health (Zator Estes, 2002). I note that a BMI of 33+ is a (UKMEC, 2016) category 1 and will pose no risk.

Her past medical history revealed she

has nil history of surgery, embolism, cardiac problems, migraines, cancer, irregular vaginal bleeding or other concern. Which would be a risk factor for considering some forms of contraception. Her medication history is Desogestrel 75 mcg, oral, daily for 5 years.

Gathering of medical history allows and informs the clinical decision making process. The relationship between the patient and the professional will be formed around the health assessment skills (Ford et al, 2005). I checked her cervical smear status and confirmed that this is negative, because this then confirms she has no current risk of cervical cancer, which would have implications when considering (UKMEC, 2016) safety categories.

The findings of the consultation and assessment were that the client is an established pill user, aware how to take the pill and is compliant and does not forget it. These are requirements and set out in guidelines Contraception - progestogen-only methods (NICE, 2015) which help establish the method is suitable. The client had no physical health problems, no allergies, no (UKMEC, 2016) concerns and I therefore determined she is safe to continue the POP. Her repeat and past medication history was also considered and confirmed as Desogestrel 75mcg daily. I utilized my present knowledge and referred to (UKMEC, 2016) guidelines. This tool allows me to confirm that the client is safe to remain on the POP.

The (Summary of Product Characteristics, 2016) Cerazette 75mcg film-coated tablet, confirms a therapeutic indication for contraception. I checked there were no contra-indications for the use of the same. I reminded the client about the effects of herbal remedies such as St Johns' wort which can interact with POP and effect the efficacy of it (Baxter 2010; Hall et al, 2003; Zhou et al, 2004).

In conclusion, following a review of the above, my clinical decision was that it was safe for her to remain on Desogestrel 75 mcg and the DMP issued a repeat prescription for Desogestrel tablets 75mcg, one tablet oral daily, 168 tablets. I reflected on local guidelines which advocate the use of Desogestrel as a generic choice for Cerazette and considered the cost for doing the same. I felt confident in my physical assessment, history taking and medication review and this informed me that Desogestrel was an effective choice of POP (Rice et al, 1999; Korver et al, 2005), for my client. I noted from her records she had been attending every 6 months for a pill check and felt it was appropriate to continue the same and good practice to review the client twice per year. I advised her if any problems she should make an appointment for a review.

My thoughts after the OSCE were that I felt under pressure and rather anxious during the process and had not expected to. (Gibbs, 1988) supports the idea of anxiety and says this is a negative but normal expected effect. I felt I utilized tools well. I felt the consultation went smoothly and the rapport was good. I recognized how the client utilized her autonomy and I utilized my accountability and professionalism. I can reflect positively on how this relationship impacted on an honest and positive consultation process for both of us, which concluded with a joint decision to repeat the prescription for a POP. My thoughts were around how the consultation process had been constructive but also a learning curve as I had undergone my fist OSCE and my communication skills were challenged into a 3-way process. This process is known as the 'dyad' and 'triad' consultation stages (Swinglehurst et al, 2014). The ''dyad" is the normal and when the 'triad' phase begins then this disturbs and challenges normal communication and I thought this was typical within the OSCE.

The patient gave simple and open verbal consent for OSCE and consultation as required and set out in (The Code for nurses and midwives, NMC, 2015). I obtained written feedback from her which was excellent and reflects a satisfied client. I learnt how the Calgary Cambridge consultation model (Silverman et al, 2013) can be beneficial during a consultation. I learnt how the 'dyad and the 'triad' phases of communication impact on practice and decisions made (Swinglehurst et al, 2014). I utilized the evidence base available to confirm the treatment was appropriate and was sure Desogestrel was the right choice of contraception for the client.

I also reflected in the patient record to ensure I was happy with my documentation and that was confirmed also, thus enabling a good medical history of events.

The portfolio also entails multiple sign offs by the Designated Medical Prescriber (DMP) who will assess you throughout your journey. You will also be required to submit a number of prescriptions and the samples can be seen later in this book. The portfolio can be concluded nicely with a written conclusion to establish the journey you have been on and to evaluate how you have changed during the time spent on the Non-Medical Prescribing course.

Conclusion

This portfolio is an honest and accurate reflection of my journey into the world of Non-Medical Prescribing. At the beginning of the journey I simply had no idea where the journey would take me and I could not envisage coming out the other end of what seemed a huge tunnel of learning and paper exercises. As I set about achieving each competence I found myself becoming more and more inquisitive and searching out the evidence why a prescription would be needed or had been given. I started to look at drugs and medicines in a different light and questions arose every day. As I started to develop my knowledge I found a new confidence within myself to discuss things around medications with patients that I had never discussed before. Today I find myself with a new confidence to challenge why prescriptions where given and what would be the benefit and risks of the same. I have read a plethora of evidence to recall in practice. At the beginning of the course I envisaged that when I completed the course I would prescribe with ease and confidence, yet this course has taught me to stop and consider all options before prescribing at all. My curiosity around drugs and to prescribe or not to prescribe will continue with me always.

Along the way, I realized many things need to be considered that I would never have stopped to think about before. I can honestly say this log of learning was my enemy at times but in the end, it became my best friend and a support mechanism to utilize in practice. This portfolio was a mystery to me 7 months ago, and I could never have contemplated that one day I would be here writing a conclusion to a learning experience which has possibly changed the way I think, practice and view prescribing and prescriptions and the responsibilities behind this forever. It gives me a great deal of satisfaction to reflect on this portfolio, which I am sure I will refer to in the future and possibly share with other Non-Medical Prescribing students also.

Reference list

Baxter, K. (2010) Stockley's drug interactions pocket companion 2010 [eBook]. London: Pharmaceutical Press.

Benagiano, G., **Primiero, F.M.** (2003) Seventy-five microgram desogestrel mini pill, a new perspective in estrogen-free contraception, **Ann N Y Acad Sci.** 2003 Nov;997:163-173

Beauchamp, T. L. & Childress, J. F. (2013) Principles of biomedical ethics, 7th edition. New York: Oxford University Press.

Bray, G.A., **Frühbeck, G.**, Ryan, D.H., (2016) Management of obesity. **Lancet.** 2016 Feb 8. pii: S0140-6736(16)00271-3. doi: 10.1016/S0140-6736(16)00271-3. [Epub ahead of print

British National Formulary (2015-2016)

Joint Formulary Committee. 70th Edition. London: British Medical Associations of Royal Pharmaceutical Society of Great Britian.

Clarke, R., Munir, R (2012) Ear, Nose and throat at a glance (eBook). Oxford: Wiley-Blackwell.

Dallosso H.M., **Eborall**, H.C., **Daly**, H., **Martin-Stacey**, L., **Speight**, J., **Realf**, K **Carey**, M.E.,

Campbell, M.J., **Dixon**, S., **Khunti**, K., **Davies**, M.J.,

Heller, S. (2012) Does self- monitoring of blood glucose as opposed to urinalysis provide additional benefit in patients newly diagnosed with type 2 diabetes receiving structured education? The DESMOND SMBG randomised controlled trial protocol, BMC Fam Pract. 2012; 13: 18. Published online 2012 Mar 14. doi: **10.1186/1471-2296-13-18**
Davies, M.J., Gray, L.J., Troughton, J., Gray, A., Tuomilehto, J., Farooqi, A., Khunt, K., Yates, T. (2016) A community based primary prevention programme for type 2 diabetes integrating identification and lifestyle intervention for prevention: the Let's Prevent Diabetes cluster randomised controlled trial. **Prev Med.** 2016 Mar;84:48-56. doi: 10.1016/j.ypmed.2015.12.012. Epub 2015 Dec 29.

Dhutia H, Sharma S (2015) Playing it safe: exercise and cardiovascular health. **Practitioner.** 2015 Oct;259(1786):15-20,

2.

Ear Care Guidance Document, (2014) Procedure for ear irrigation, aural toilet, ear instrumentation and microsuction. The Rotherham NHS Foundation Trust, Rotherham, UK

Epstein B, **Turner M**.(2015) The Nursing Code of Ethics: Its Value, Its History, **Online J** Issues **Nurs.** 2015 May 31;20(2):4.

Farokhzadian,J., **Nayeri, N.D.**, **Borhani, F.**, **Zare, M.R**. (2015) Nurse leaders' Attitudes, Self-Efficacy and training Needs for Implementing Evidence-Based Practice: Is It Time for a Change toward Safe Care? **Br J Med Med Res.** 2015;7(8):662-671. Epub 2015 Mar 17.

Grimes, R.T .,**Bennett, K.**, **Canavan, R.**, **Tilson, L.**, **Henman, M.C**. (2016) The impact of initial antidiabetic agent and use of monitoring agents on prescription costs in newly treated type 2 diabetes: A retrospective cohort analysis. **Diabetes Res Clin Pract.** 2016 Mar;113:152-9. doi: 10.1016/j.diabres.2015.12.020. Epub 2016 Jan 13.

Hall, S.D., **Wang, Z.**, **Huang, S.M.**, **Hamman, M.A.**,**Vasavada, N. Adigun, A.Q.**, **Hilligoss, J.K.**, **Miller, M.**, **Gorski, J.C**. (2003), The Interaction between St Johns' wort and an oral contraceptive,.**Clin Pharmacol Ther.** 2003 Dec;74(6):525-35.

Holt, T. A., Kumar, S. & Watkins, P. J. (2010) ABC of diabetes, 6th edition [eBook]. Oxford: Wiley-Blackwell.

Hull and East Riding Prescribing Committee (2013) Good Practice in Self-Blood Glucose Monitoring (SBGM) Type 1 and Type 2 Diabetes Guidance for Health Care Professionals. Available Online: www. **www.hey.nhs.uk/herpc/prescribing-guidelines.htm** (Accessed on 24th March 2016

Hull and East Riding Prescribing Committee (2015) Algorithm for the Treatment of Type 2 Diabetes Mellitus. Available Online: Available Online: **www.hey.nhs.uk/herpc/guidlines/algorithmType2DiabetesMellitus** (Accessed Online 1st February 2016)

Johnson, M. T. (2011) The diversity code: unlock the secrets to making differences work in the real world [eBook]. New York: AMACOM, American Management Association.

Kamarudin, G., Penn J., **Chaar**, B., **Moles**, R. (2013) Educational interventions to improve prescribing competency: a systematic review, BMJ Open. 2013; 3(8): e003291. Published online 2013 Aug 29. doi: **10.1136/bmjopen-2013-003291**

Klonoff, D.C., **Blonde**, L., **Chacra**, A.R., **Charpentier**, G., **Colagiuri**, S., **George Dailey**, **Gabbay**, R.A., **Heinemann**, L., **Kerr**, D., **Nicolucci**, A., **Polonsky**, W., **Schnell**, O.,**Robert Vigersky**, R.M., **Yale**,

J.F (2011) Consensus Report: The Current Role of Self-Monitoring of Blood Glucose in Non-Insulin-Treated Type 2 Diabetes, J Diabetes Sci Technol. 2011 Nov; 5(6): 1529–1548. Published online 2011 Nov 1.

Kogan, M., Redfern, S. J. & Kober, A. (1995) Making use of clinical audit: a guide to practice in the health professions. Buckingham: Open University Press.

Korver, T., Klipping, C., Duijkers I, Van Osta, G., Dieben, T. (2005) Maintenance of ovulation inhibition with the 75-microg desogestrel-only Contraceptive pill (Cerazette) after scheduled 12-h delays in tablet intake. **Contraception.** 2005 Jan;71(1):8-13.

Medicines and Healthcare Products Regulatory Agency (2014) Combined hormonal contraceptives and venous thromboembolism: review confirms risk is small. Available online: **www.gov.uk/medicines-and-healthcare-products-regulatory-agency** (Accessed 21st Match 2016)

Morrell, C. & Harvey, G. (1999) The clinical audit handbook: improving the quality of health care. London: Baillière Tindall.

National Institute for Health and Care Excellence (2015) Type 2 Diabetes in Adults; Management, [NG28]. Available Online: **www.nice.org.uk/guidance/ng28 Accessed 22nd March 2016**

National Institute for Health and Care Excellence (2015) Contraception

Progestogen–Only Contraception Methods, Published date February 2015. Available Online: **www.nice.org.uk** (accessed 1st March 2016)

National Institute for Health Care Excellence (2016) MiniMed 640G system with Smart Guard for managing blood glucose levels in people with type 1 diabetes. Available Online: **www.nice.org.uk/advice/mib51/chapter/Introduction** (Accessed 23rd March 2016)

Neighbour, R. (2005) The inner consultation: how to develop an effective and intuitive consulting style, 2nd edition. Abingdon: Radcliffe.

Nice (2009) The management of type 2 diabetes, DOH, London, UK

Orem, D. E. (1995). Nursing: concepts of practice. 5th ed. St. Louis: Mosby.

Osei, E., Fonville, S., Zandbergen, A.A., Koudstaal, P.J., Dippel, D.W., Den Hertog, H.M (2016) Glucose in prediabetic and diabetic range and outcome after stroke. Available Online: **www.onlinelibrary.wiley.com/doi/10.1111/ane.12577/references** (Accessed Online 2nd February 2016

Parkin, C.G., **Jaime A. Davidson**, J.A. (2009) Value of Self-Monitoring Blood Glucose Pattern Analysis in Improving Diabetes Outcomes, J Diabetes Sci Technol. 2009 May; 3(3): 500–508. Published online 2009 May.

Rice, C., Killick., S., Dieben, T., Coelingh

Bennick, H., (1999) A comparison of the inhibition of ovulation achieved by desogestrel 75 µg and levonorgestrel 30 µg daily. *HUM REPROD* 1999; **14**(4): 982–985.

Rosen, M. (1979) The Sunday Times thalidomide case. London: Writers and Scholars Education Trust.

Sidney, S., Cheetham, T.C., Connell, F.A., Ouellet-Hellstrom, R., Graham, D.J,., Davis, D., Sorel, M., Quesenberry, C.P., Jr, Cooper, W.O. (2012) Recent combined hormonal contraceptives (CHCs) and the risk of thromboembolism and other cardiovascular events in new users, **Contraception.** 2013 Jan;87(1):93-100. doi: 10.1016/j.contraception.2012.09.015. Epub 2012 Oct 19.

Stegeman, B.H., DeBastos, M., Rosendaal, F.R., Van Helmerhorst, F.M., Stijnen, T., Dekkers, O.M. (2014) Different combined oral contraceptives and the risk of venous thrombosis: systematic review and network meta-analysis. **BMJ.** 2013 Sep 12;347 f5298. doi: 10.1136/bmj.f5298.

Summary of Products Characteristics (2015) Desogestrel 75 microgram Film-coated Tablets. Available online: **www.medicines.org.uk/emc/history/30384** (Accessed 21st March 2016)

Unwin D., Tobin, S. (2015) A patient request for some "deprescribing". **BMJ.** 2015 Aug 3;351:h4023. doi:

10.1136/bmj.h4023.

Vistisen, D., **Andersen, G.S.**, **Hansen, C.S.**, **Hulman, A.**, **Henriksen, J.E.**, **Beck-Nielsen, H.**, **Jørgensen, M.E.**, (2016) Prediction of First Cardiovascular Disease Event in Type 1 Diabetes: The Steno T1 Risk Engine. Circulation 2016 Feb 17. pii: CIRCULATIONAHA.115.018844. [Epub ahead of print]

Waite, M. & Keenan, J. (2010) CPD for non-medical prescribers: a practical guide. Chichester: Wiley-Blackwell.

Zhou, S., **Chan, E.**, **Pan, S.Q.**, **Huang, M.**, **Lee, E.J.**, (2004) Phamacokinetic interactions of drugs St John's wort, **J Psychopharmacol.** 2004 Jun;18(2):262-7

Ziller, M., Ziller, V., Haas, G., Rex, J., Kostev, K. (2013) of venous thrombosis in users of hormonal contraceptives in German gynaecological practices: a patient database analysis. **Arch Gynecol Obstet.** 2014 Feb;289(2):413-9. doi: 10.1007/s00404-013-2983-9. Epub 2013 Aug 4.

Printed in Great Britain
by Amazon